TYPE 2 DIABETES DIET COOKBOOK 2024

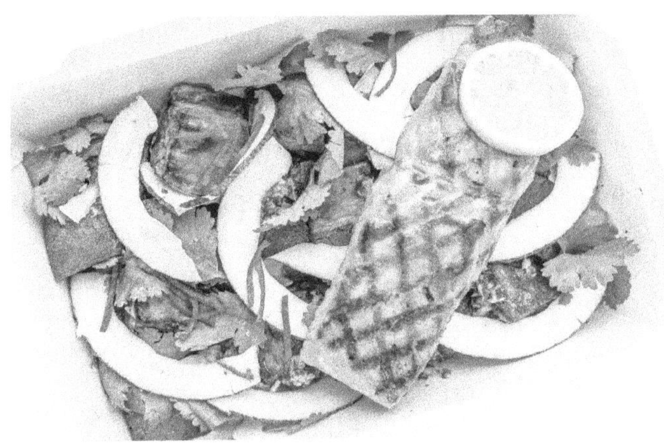

Discover the transformative power of healthful, delicious dishes expertly developed to help you on your path to wellness

Misty J. Font

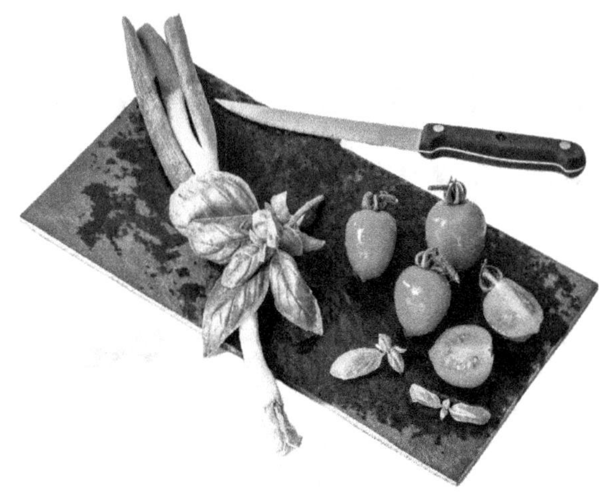

Table of contents

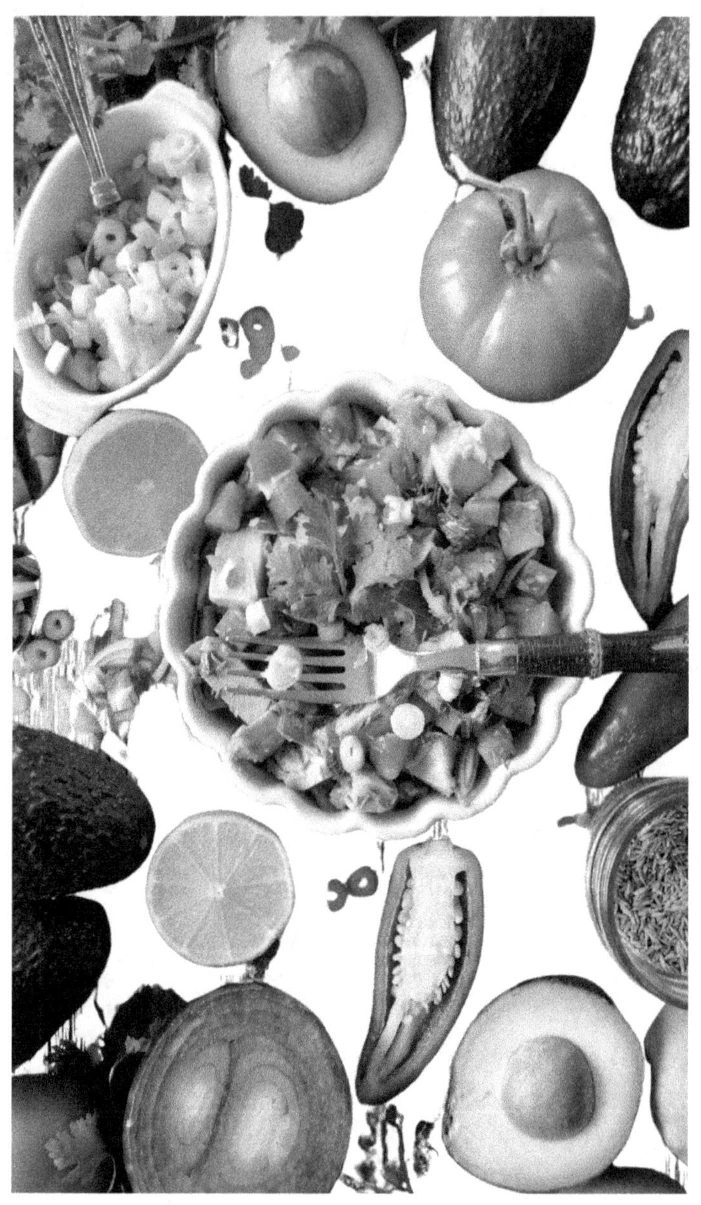

CHAPTER 1:
INTRODUCTION

John has always been a man of habit. Every morning, he'd get up with the sun, make a pot of coffee, and sit at his kitchen table, scanning the newspaper while sipping his caffeine fix. However, on one of these perfectly routine mornings, John's life took a surprising turn.

As John reached for the sugar bowl to sweeten his coffee, his palm trembled uncontrollably. He dismissed it, attributing it to exhaustion following a rough night's sleep. However, as the days went, his symptoms deteriorated. Fatigue lingered like an unwanted shadow, and his vision appeared to blur around the edges. Concerned, John set up an appointment with his doctor.

Following a series of testing, John received a devastating diagnosis: Type 2 Diabetes. He was stunned. How does this happen? He took pride in his healthy lifestyle, but his doctor stated that genetics, combined with poor eating habits over the years, had caught up with him.

When confronted with the truth of his illness, John understood he needed to make a difference. But where do I start? The world of diabetes treatment seems overwhelming, with contradicting information and complicated diet planning. Feeling overwhelmed, John turned to the only constancy in his life: books.

While browsing the shelves of his local bookshop, John came across a beacon of hope: the Type 2 Diabetes Diet Cookbook. He browsed through its pages, each one loaded with colorful photos of tasty, diabetes-friendly meals. It claimed simple recipes made with healthful ingredients that would help to balance blood sugar levels and enhance general health.

With the cookbook in hand, John set off on a path of transformation. Gone were the days of easy foods and sugary treats. Instead, he adopted a new eating style that emphasized fresh produce, lean proteins, and entire grains.

Armed with his newfound knowledge, John returned to the kitchen with renewed zeal. He chopped, sautéed, and simmered his way through the cookbook, taking pleasure in the smells of herbs and spices as they danced in the air. Each meal became a gastronomic experience, demonstrating his determination to restore his health.

However, the road to rehabilitation was not without its hurdles. Temptation lingered around every corner, talking seductively about fast food and sumptuous treats. Nonetheless, John stayed strong in his commitment, drawing strength from the good changes he could already sense taking root in his body.

As the weeks grew into months, John's efforts began to pay off. His energy levels increased, and his waistline gradually began to decrease. Most importantly, his blood sugar levels stabilized and no longer fluctuated wildly like a pendulum.

John's progress encouraged him to share his story with friends and family, inspiring them to take control of their own health. They shared recipes and tales, celebrating minor victories along the way.

So, armed with only a cookbook and a drive to thrive, John set off on a quest of self-discovery. Through the power of food, he discovered not just health but also a renewed sense of purpose. For John, the Type 2 Diabetes Diet Cookbook was more than just a compilation of recipes; it was a road map to a better, healthier future.

Understanding Type II Diabetes

What is Type 2 diabetes?

Type 2 diabetes, often known as adult-onset diabetes, is a chronic metabolic condition characterized by high blood sugar (glucose). Unlike Type 1 Diabetes, which occurs when the body fails to create enough insulin, Type 2 Diabetes occurs when the body's cells fail to respond appropriately to insulin, resulting in an accumulation of glucose in the bloodstream.

Causes and Risk Factors

The causes of Type 2 Diabetes are complex, with hereditary and lifestyle factors playing important roles. The key risk factors include family history, obesity, a sedentary lifestyle, poor eating habits, and advanced age. Furthermore, certain ethnic groups, including African Americans, Hispanics, Native Americans, and Asian Americans, are more likely to develop Type 2 diabetes.

complications of type 2 diabetes

Untreated or poorly controlled Type 2 Diabetes can cause a slew of problems that impact many organs and systems in the body. Uncontrolled blood sugar levels have a wide range of consequences for overall health, including cardiovascular disease, neuropathy, nephropathy, and retinopathy, as well as a higher risk of stroke, peripheral vascular disease, and even foot issues.

The Role of Diet in Managing Type 2 Diabetes

Despite the difficulties of Type 2 Diabetes therapy, nutrition emerges as a critical component of good control and prevention. Individuals with Type 2 Diabetes can control their blood sugar levels, enhance insulin sensitivity, manage their weight, and reduce their risk of complications by choosing wise food choices.

Tips for Managing Type 2 Diabetes Through Diet

Navigating the panorama of food options with Type 2 Diabetes can be challenging, but it doesn't have to be. Here are some practical recommendations that will help you on your quest to improved health:

Focus on full, unprocessed foods: Include plenty of fruits, vegetables, lean proteins, and whole grains in your meals. These foods are high in critical nutrients, fiber, and antioxidants, which promote general health and help regulate blood sugar levels.

Watch your carbs: Limit your carbohydrate intake and choose complex carbohydrates with a low glycemic index, such as whole grains, legumes, and non-starchy vegetables. These carbs breakdown more slowly, causing moderate blood sugar changes.

Pay attention to portion proportions to avoid overeating and keep a healthy weight. To avoid consuming too many calories, use smaller plates, calculate your quantities, and eat mindfully.

Limit your use of sugary beverages, processed foods, and sweets that contain added sugars and refined carbohydrates. These foods can produce rapid blood sugar increases, which can lead to insulin resistance over time.

Stay hydrated: Drink plenty of water throughout the day to keep your body hydrated and functioning properly. To add variety, avoid sugary drinks and instead drink water, herbal teas, or sparkling water flavored with a touch of citrus.

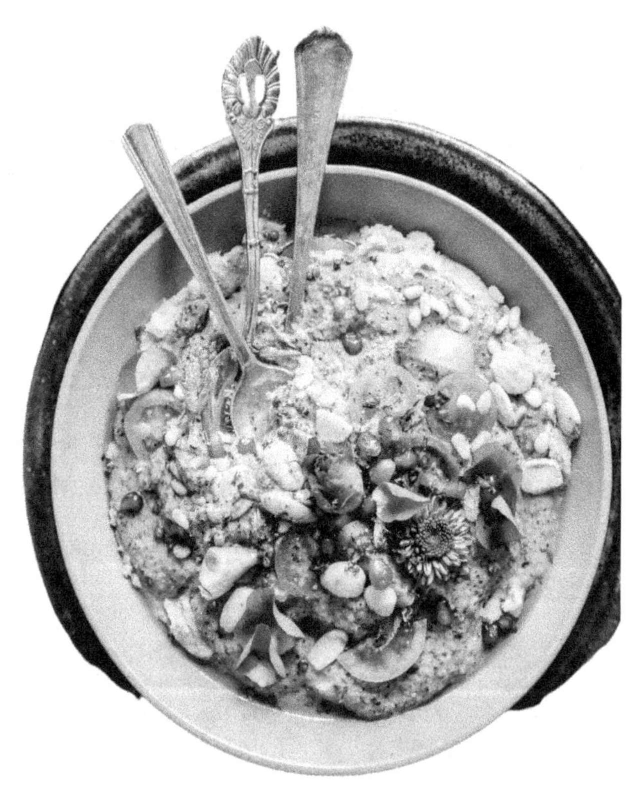

Chapter 2: The Fundamentals of A Type 2 Diabetes Diet

Welcome to part 2 of our complete guide on managing Type 2 Diabetes with Diet. In this chapter, we establish the framework for developing a diabetes-friendly diet that promotes blood sugar stability, aids in weight management, and improves overall health. Let's go over the principles of a Type 2 Diabetes diet and equip you with the knowledge and skills you need to succeed.

Basics of a Diabetes-Friendly Diet

A diabetes-friendly diet is based on concepts that prioritize nutrient-dense, whole foods while limiting the consumption of processed and refined items. Fruits, vegetables, lean proteins, and healthy fats are the foundation of a balanced food plan for those with type 2 diabetes. By focusing on high-quality, nutrient-dense foods, you can improve your health and blood sugar control.

Carbohydrate Counting and Glycemic Index

Carbohydrate counting and understanding the glycemic index (GI) are critical strategies for regulating blood sugar levels in people with Type 2 Diabetes. Carbohydrates have the greatest impact on blood glucose levels, thus it is critical to monitor and restrict your intake. You may make informed decisions about which carbs to include in your diet and in what quantities if you are familiar with the glycemic index, which evaluates carbohydrates based on their influence on blood sugar.

Portion Control & Meal Timing

Portion control and meal timing are critical in maintaining blood sugar levels and increasing satiety throughout the day. By eating balanced meals at regular intervals and limiting portion sizes, you can avoid blood sugar spikes and crashes while maintaining consistent energy levels. Furthermore, paying attention to meal scheduling, such as spacing meals evenly throughout the day and avoiding heavy meals late at night, can assist improve glycemic control and metabolic health.

Create a Balanced Plate

Creating a balanced plate is a simple but effective way to improve nutrition and blood sugar control. Aim to fill half of your plate with non-starchy veggies, one-quarter with lean protein, and one-quarter with whole grains or starchy vegetables. Incorporating a diversity of colors, textures, and flavors not only improves the visual attractiveness of your meals, but also assures a wide range of nutrients to support maximum health and vitality.

Understanding Food Labels

Navigating food labels can be difficult, but understanding how to decipher them is critical for making informed eating decisions. When reading food labels, consider portion sizes, total carbohydrate content, fiber content, and added sugars. To help you manage your diabetes, look for items that have fewer added sugars, more fiber, and whole food ingredients.

Chapter 3: Breakfasts for Healthy Blood Sugar

Berry Almond Chia Pudding

Berry Almond Chia Pudding is a creamy and delightful recipe with brilliant tastes of fresh berries and crunchy almonds. It's the ideal way to start the day on a healthful note, thanks to its high fiber content and beneficial fats.

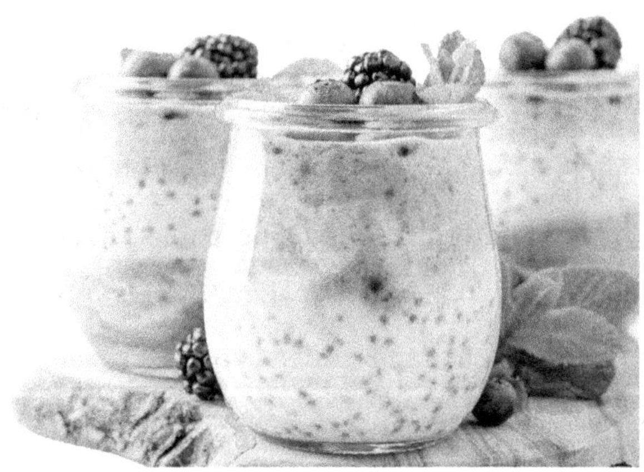

Serving Size: Two servings

Prep time: 5 minutes.

Cooking time: 0 minutes.

Ingredients:

- 1/4 cup of chia seeds.
- 1 cup of unsweetened almond milk.
- 1/2 cup mixed berries (strawberries, blueberries and raspberries)
- 2 tablespoons sliced almonds.
- 1 tablespoon of honey or maple syrup (optional).

Instructions:

1. a mixing bowl, add chia seeds and almond milk. Stir well to properly distribute the chia seeds.
2. Cover the bowl and chill for at least 2 hours, preferably overnight, to allow the chia seeds to absorb the liquid and thicken into a pudding-like texture.
3. Before serving, divide the chia pudding among individual bowls or jars.
4. Top each plate with a mix of berries and chopped almonds.
5. Drizzle with honey or maple syrup as desired.

6. Enjoy immediately or refrigerate leftovers for up to three days.

Veggie Egg Muffins

Veggie Egg Muffins are a low-carb breakfast option that includes colorful vegetables and protein-rich eggs. They're ideal for meal preparation and can be personalized with your preferred vegetables and seasonings.

Serving size: six muffins.
Prep time: 10 minutes.
Cook time: 20 minutes.

Ingredients:

- six eggs.
- 1/4 cup sliced bell peppers (red, green, and yellow).
- 1/4 cup chopped tomatoes.
- 1/4 cup chopped spinach.
- 1/4 cup chopped onions.

- 1/4 cup shredded cheese (cheddar or mozzarella)
- Add salt and pepper to taste.

Instructions:

1. Preheat the oven to 350° Fahrenheit (175° Celsius). Grease a muffin tray or use muffin liners.
2. In a mixing bowl, whisk the eggs until well combined. Season with salt and pepper to taste.
3. Divide the diced vegetables evenly into the muffin cups.
4. Pour the beaten eggs over the vegetables, filling each muffin cup 3/4 full.
5. Sprinkle grated cheese over the top of each muffin.
6. Bake in the preheated oven for 18-20 minutes, or until the egg muffins are firm and faintly brown on top.
7. Remove from the oven and allow it cool for a few minutes before serving.
8. Enjoy warm or refrigerate leftovers in an airtight jar for up to three days.

Greek Yogurt Parfait

Greek Yogurt Parfait is a protein-rich breakfast option that is quick and easy to make. It's a filling and healthful way to start the day, with creamy Greek yogurt, fresh berries, and crunchy granola on top.

Serving Size: One parfait.
Prep time: 5 minutes.
Cooking time: 0 minutes.

Ingredients:

- 1/2 cup of Greek yogurt.
- 1/4 cup mixed berries (strawberries, blueberries and raspberries)
- 2 tbsp granola.
- One teaspoon of honey or maple syrup (optional)

Instructions:

1. In a glass or bowl, layer half of the Greek yogurt.
2. Place half of the mixed berries on top of the yogurt.

3. Sprinkle with one tablespoon of granola.

4. Repeat the layers with the remaining yogurt, berries, and granola.

5. Drizzle with honey or maple syrup as desired.

6. Serve immediately and enjoy this protein-rich parfait.

Avocado toast with poached eggs

Avocado toast with a freshly poached egg is a simple and fulfilling breakfast option that takes only a few minutes to prepare. The creamy avocado spread on whole-grain bread has healthy fats and fiber, while the poached egg provides protein for a balanced start to the day.

Serving Size: One serving

Prep time: 5 minutes.

Cook time: 5 minutes.

Ingredients:

- 1 piece of healthy grain bread and 1/2 ripe avocado.

- 1 egg

- Add salt and pepper to taste.

- Red pepper flakes (optional).

- Chopped fresh herbs are optional.

Instructions:

1. Toast the whole grain bread till golden brown.

2. While the bread is toasting, mash the avocado in a small bowl and season with salt, pepper, and red pepper flakes, if desired.

3. Poach an egg: Heat a pot of water to a low simmer. Crack one egg into a small bowl or ramekin. Create a gently swirl in the simmering water with a spoon, then delicately slip the egg into the center. Cook for 3-4 minutes to make a gently poached egg.

4. With a slotted spoon, remove the poached egg and place it on a paper towel to drain any extra water.

5. Spread the mashed avocado on the toasted bread.

6. Top with the poached egg and, if preferred, add more salt, pepper, and chopped fresh herbs.

7. Serve immediately and enjoy a quick and nutritious breakfast.

Overnight oats

Preparing overnight oats ahead of time is a convenient and versatile breakfast option for hectic mornings. Simply combine oats, your preferred milk, yogurt, and toppings, and refrigerate overnight for a tasty and nutritious breakfast the next day.

Serving Size: One serving

Prep time: 5 minutes.

Cooking time: 0 minutes.

Ingredients:

- 1/2 cup of rolled oats.
- 1/2 cup unsweetened almond milk (or any milk you want)
- 1/4 cup Greek yogurt.
- 1 tablespoon of chia seeds.
- 1/2 teaspoon of vanilla extract.

- 1 tablespoon of honey or maple syrup (optional).
- Toppings include sliced bananas, berries, almonds, seeds, nut butter, and shredded coconut.

Instructions:

1. In a mason jar or airtight container, combine the rolled oats, almond milk, Greek yogurt, chia seeds, vanilla extract, and honey or maple syrup, if desired. Stir thoroughly to mix.
2. Toppings include sliced bananas, berries, almonds, seeds, and nut butter.
3. Cover the jar or container and refrigerate overnight, or at least 4 hours, to let the oats soak and soften.
4. In the morning, stir the overnight oats and add extra milk if needed for a thinner consistency.
5. Enjoy cold straight from the fridge, or heat in the microwave for a warm breakfast.
6. Customize with different toppings each time for diversity, and eat these make-ahead overnight oats all week.

7. These breakfast recipes are intended to not only fuel your body but also maintain stable blood sugar levels and deliver long-lasting energy throughout the day.

8. Whether you want a high-fiber alternative, a low-carb supper, or a quick and easy recipe for hectic mornings, there is something for everyone.

9. Begin your day right with these delicious, diabetes-friendly breakfasts!

Quinoa Breakfast Bowl

Quinoa Breakfast Bowl is a high-protein and fiber-rich dish with almonds. Topped with fresh fruits and a drizzle of honey, it's a delightful and nutritious way to start the day.

Serving Size: Two servings

Prep time: 10 minutes.

Cook time: 15 minutes.

Ingredients:

- 1/2 cup quinoa, rinsed.

- 1 cup water.

- 1/2 teaspoon of cinnamon.

- 1/4 cup chopped nuts (such as almonds, walnuts, or pecans)

- 1/2 cup sliced strawberries.

- 1/2 cup blueberries.

- Two teaspoons of honey or maple syrup

Instructions:

- Heat water in a small pot until it boils. Add the quinoa and turn the heat down to low.

- Cover and simmer for 12-15 minutes, or until the quinoa is cooked and the water has been absorbed.

- Fluff the quinoa with a fork and add the cinnamon.

- Divide the cooked quinoa across serving bowls.

- Top each bowl with chopped nuts, cut strawberries, and blueberries.

- Drizzle with either honey or maple syrup.

- Enjoy this filling, high-fiber breakfast bowl while still warm.

Spinach and Feta Crustless Quiche

This crustless quiche with spinach, feta cheese, and eggs is a low-carb, protein-rich breakfast choice. It's ideal for meal prep and can be eaten warm or cold, making it a versatile and practical option for busy mornings.

Serving Size: Four servings
Prep time: 10 minutes.
Cook time: 30 minutes.

Ingredients:
- Six big eggs.
- 1/2 cup milk (unsweetened almond milk)
- 2 cups fresh spinach, chopped.
- 1/4 cup crumbled feta cheese.
- 1/4 teaspoon of garlic powder.
- Add salt and pepper to taste.

Instructions:

1. Preheat the oven to 375° Fahrenheit (190° Celsius). Grease a 9-inch pie pan or baking dish.
2. In a mixing bowl, whisk together the eggs and milk until thoroughly blended.
3. Combine the chopped spinach, crumbled feta cheese, garlic powder, salt, and pepper.
4. Pour the egg mixture into the prepared pie dish.
5. Bake for 25-30 minutes, or until the quiche has set and turned golden brown on top.
6. Remove from the oven and allow it cool for a few minutes before cutting.
7. Serve warm or store leftovers for later use.

Cottage Cheese Pancakes

Cottage cheese, eggs, and whole wheat flour combine to make these fluffy and protein-packed pancakes. Served with fresh fruit and a sprinkle of honey, they're a delightful and nutritious way to start the day with a surge of energy.

Servings: 2 (4 pancakes)

Prep time: 10 minutes.

Cooking time: 10 minutes.

Ingredients:

- One cup cottage cheese.
- Two huge eggs.
- 1/2 cup of whole wheat flour.
- 1 teaspoon of baking powder.
- 1/4 teaspoon cinnamon.
- 1/4 teaspoon of vanilla extract.
- Fresh fruit and honey to serve.

Instructions:

1. In a blender or food processor, combine cottage cheese, eggs, whole wheat flour, baking powder, cinnamon, and vanilla extract. Blend until smooth.

2. Heat a nonstick skillet or griddle over medium heat, then lightly coat with cooking spray or oil.

3. Pour roughly 1/4 cup pancake batter into the skillet for each pancake.

4. Cook for 2-3 minutes, or until bubbles appear on the surface of the pancakes and the edges start to firm.

5. Flip the pancakes and cook for another 1-2 minutes on the other side, or until golden brown and fully cooked.

6. Serve the pancakes warm, topped with fresh fruit and honey.

Peanut Butter Banana Smoothie

This Peanut Butter Banana Smoothie combines peanut butter, banana, Greek yogurt, and almond milk for a quick and easy breakfast option. It's a tasty way to power your day, with plenty of protein and potassium.

Serving Size: One serving

Prep time: 5 minutes.

Cooking time: 0 minutes.

Ingredients:

- 1 peeled and frozen ripe banana.

- 1 tablespoon of peanut butter.

- 1/2 cup Greek yogurt.

- 1/2 cup unsweetened almond milk (or any milk you want)

- 1/4 teaspoon cinnamon.

- 1/2 cup of ice cubes (optional)

Instructions:

1. To make the smoothie, blend frozen bananas, peanut butter, Greek yogurt, almond milk, cinnamon, and optional ice cubes.

2. Blend until smooth and creamy, adding additional almond milk as needed to achieve the desired consistency.

3. Pour the smoothie into a glass and serve it immediately.

Egg Muffin Cups With Turkey and Vegetables

These egg muffin cups are filled with lean turkey, colorful vegetables, and eggs, making them a protein-rich and convenient breakfast alternative. They are ideal for meal prep because they can be prepared ahead of time and eaten throughout the week for a quick and handy breakfast on the run.

Serving size: six muffin cups.

Prep time: 10 minutes.

Cook time: 20 minutes.

Ingredients:

- Six big eggs.
- 1/4 cup sliced bell peppers (red, green, and yellow).
- 1/4 cup chopped tomatoes.
- 1/4 cup chopped spinach.
- 1/4 cup chopped onions.
- 1/4 cup diced turkey breast, cooked
- Add salt and pepper to taste.

Instructions:

1. Preheat the oven to 375° Fahrenheit (190° Celsius).

2. Grease a muffin tray or use muffin liners.

3. In a mixing bowl, whisk the eggs until well combined.

4. Season with salt and pepper to taste.

5. Divide the diced vegetables and turkey equally among the muffin cups.

6. Pour the beaten eggs over the vegetables and turkey, filling each muffin cup 3/4 full.

7. Bake in the preheated oven for 18-20 minutes, or until the egg muffin cups are firm and gently brown on top.

8. Remove from the oven and allow it cool for a few minutes before serving.

9. Enjoy warm or store leftovers for later.

Chapter 4: Nutritious Lunches for Stable Energy

Grilled Chicken with Quinoa Salad

This colorful salad features succulent grilled chicken, fluffy quinoa, and sharp veggies mixed in a zesty lemon vinaigrette. It's a refreshing and filling lunch option that you may enjoy all year.

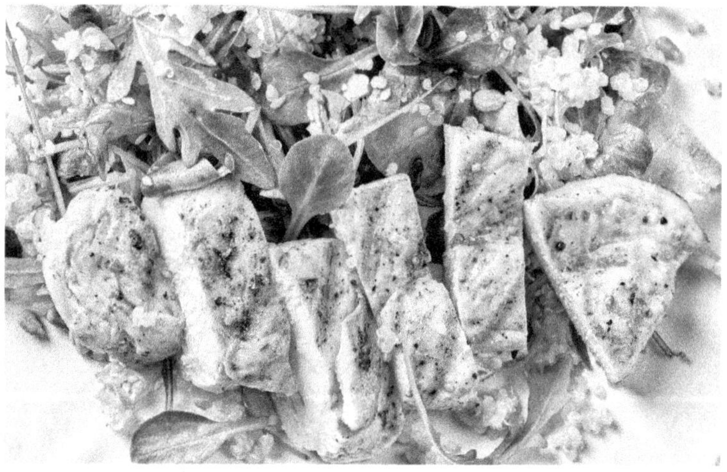

Serving Size: Two servings

Prep time: 15 minutes.

Cook time: 15 minutes.

Ingredients:

- 2 boneless and skinless chicken breasts.
- Ingredients: 1/2 cup rinsed quinoa, 1 cup halved cherry tomatoes, and 1 sliced cucumber.
- 1/4 red onion, thinly sliced
- 2 cups of mixed greens (spinach, arugula, or kale).
- 1/4 cup freshly chopped herbs (parsley, basil, or cilantro)
- 2 tablespoons olive oil.
- 1 tablespoon of lemon juice.
- 1 teaspoon Dijon mustard.
- Add salt and pepper to taste.

Instructions:

1. Preheat the grill or grill pan to medium-high heat. Season the chicken breasts with salt and pepper.
2. Grill the chicken for 6-8 minutes per side, or until well done and no longer pink in the center. Remove from the grill and allow to rest for a few minutes before slicing.

3. In a small saucepan, heat 1 cup of water to a boil. Add the quinoa and turn the heat down to low. Cover and simmer for 12-15 minutes, or until the quinoa is cooked and the water has been absorbed. Fluff with a fork and set aside to cool.

4. In a large mixing bowl, add the cooked quinoa, cherry tomatoes, cucumber, red onion, mixed greens, and freshly chopped herbs.

5. In a separate small bowl, combine the olive oil, lemon juice, Dijon mustard, salt, and pepper to make the vinaigrette.

6. Pour the vinaigrette over the salad and toss to coat evenly.

7. Divide the salad into individual bowls and top with sliced grilled chicken.

8. Serve immediately and enjoy this tasty and nutritious grilled chicken and quinoa salad.

Turkey avocado wrap

This turkey avocado wrap contains lean protein, healthy fats, and crisp vegetables, making it a nutritious and diabetes-friendly lunch option. It's ideal for snacking on the go or packing for work or school.

Serving Size: One wrap.

Prep time: 10 minutes.

Cooking time: 0 minutes.

Ingredients:

- One whole wheat or low-carb tortilla.
- 3 slices of deli turkey breast.
- 1/4 avocado, thinly sliced
- 1/4 cup shredded lettuce.
- 1/4 cup sliced cucumber.
- One spoonful hummus or mustard
- Add salt and pepper to taste.

Instructions:

1. Place the tortilla flat on a clean surface.
2. Spread hummus or mustard equally on the tortilla.

3. Place the deli turkey breast, avocado slices, shredded lettuce, and sliced cucumber in the center of the tortilla.

4. Season with salt and pepper to taste.

5. Fold in the tortilla's sides and roll it up tightly from the bottom to form a wrap.

6. Cut the wrap in half diagonally and serve immediately, or wrap it tightly in foil or parchment paper for later consumption.

Quinoa Veggie Buddha Bowl

Quinoa Veggie Buddha Bowl is a nutritious lunch option featuring quinoa, roasted veggies, and avocado. It's a balanced lunch that will keep you energized and satisfied all day.

Serving Size: Two servings
Prep time: 15 minutes.
Cook time: 20 minutes.

Ingredients:

- 1 cup washed quinoa.
- 2 cups mixed vegetables (bell peppers, broccoli, carrots, zucchini), chopped
- 1 tablespoon of olive oil.
- 1 teaspoon of garlic powder.
- Add salt and pepper to taste.
- One avocado, sliced
- 2 tablespoons hummus or tahini.
- Fresh lemon slices to serve

Instructions:

1. Preheat the oven to 400 °F (200 °C). Line a baking sheet with parchment paper.
2. In a small saucepan, heat 2 cups of water to a boil. Add the quinoa and turn the heat down to low. Cover and let simmer for 15 minutes, or until the quinoa is cooked and the water has been absorbed. Fluff with a fork and set aside to cool.
3. Toss the mixed veggies with olive oil, garlic powder, salt, and pepper until well covered.
4. Place the seasoned vegetables in a single layer on the prepared baking sheet.

5. Roast the vegetables in a warm oven for 15-20 minutes, or until soft and gently browned.

6. To make the Buddha bowls, divide the cooked quinoa and roasted vegetables between two bowls.

7. Top each bowl with slices of avocado and a dollop of hummus or tahini.

8. Serve with fresh lemon wedges to squeeze over the dishes just before eating.

Mediterranean Chickpea Salad

Mediterranean Chickpea Salad is a convenient lunch alternative for busy days at work or school. It's a filling breakfast with enough of protein, fiber, and flavor to keep you nourished and focused.

Serving Size: Two servings
Prep time: 10 minutes.
Cooking time: 0 minutes.

Ingredients:

- 1 (15 ounce) can of chickpeas, drained and rinsed

- To prepare, halve 1 cup cherry tomatoes and cube 1/2 cucumber.

- 1/4 cup diced red onion.

- 1/4 cup chopped fresh parsley.

- 2 tablespoons of crumbled feta cheese.

- 2 tablespoons of extra virgin olive oil.

- 1 tablespoon of red wine vinegar.

- 1 teaspoon of dried oregano.

- Add salt and pepper to taste.

- Serve with pita bread or whole grain crackers.

Instructions:

1. In a large mixing basin, mix together the chickpeas, cherry tomatoes, cucumber, red onion, parsley, and feta cheese.

2. In a small mixing bowl, combine the olive oil, red wine vinegar, dried oregano, salt, and pepper to prepare the dressing.

3. Pour the dressing over the chickpea salad and toss to coat evenly.

4. Divide the salad into individual containers for convenient transportation.

5. For a balanced and portable lunch, pair each serving with pita bread or whole-grain crackers.

Greek Chickpea Salad

This Greek-inspired chickpea salad is full of Mediterranean flavors and brilliant colors. It's a filling and nutritious lunch full of protein, fiber, and healthy fats.

Serving Size: Two servings
Prep time: 15 minutes.
Cooking time: 0 minutes.

Ingredients:

- 1 (15 ounce) can of chickpeas, drained and rinsed
- To prepare, halve 1 cup cherry tomatoes and cube 1/2 cucumber.
- 1/4 cup diced red onion.
- 1/4 cup chopped Kalamata olives

- 1/4 cup crumbled feta cheese.

- 2 tablespoons of extra virgin olive oil.

- 1 tablespoon of red wine vinegar.

- 1 teaspoon of dried oregano.

- Add salt and pepper to taste.

- Fresh parsley for garnish (optional)

Instructions:

1. In a large mixing basin, mix together the chickpeas, cherry tomatoes, cucumber, red onion, kalamata olives, and feta cheese.

2. In a small mixing bowl, combine the olive oil, red wine vinegar, dried oregano, salt, and pepper to prepare the dressing.

3. Pour the dressing over the chickpea salad and toss to coat evenly.

4. Garnish with fresh parsley before serving.

5. Divide the salad into individual bowls and enjoy this delicious Greek chickpea salad.

Hummus Vegetable Wrap

This hummus veggie wrap is a filling and nutritious lunch alternative. It's simple to customize with your favorite vegetables and hummus flavors for unlimited possibilities.

Serving Size: One wrap.

Prep time: 10 minutes.

Cooking time: 0 minutes.

Ingredients:

- One whole wheat or low-carb tortilla.
- 2 tablespoons hummus (flavor of your choosing)
- 1/4 cup shredded carrots.
- 1/4 cup of thinly sliced cucumber.
- 1/4 cup young spinach leaves.
- 1/4 avocado, sliced
- Add salt and pepper to taste.

Instructions:

1. Place the tortilla flat on a clean surface.

2. Spread the hummus evenly on the tortilla.

3. Spread the shredded carrots, sliced cucumber, baby spinach leaves, and sliced avocado along the center of the tortilla.

4. Season with salt and pepper to taste.

5. Fold in the tortilla's sides and roll it up tightly from the bottom to form a wrap.

6. Cut the wrap in half diagonally and serve immediately, or wrap it tightly in foil or parchment paper for later consumption.

Butternut Squash Soup

This creamy and cozy butternut squash soup is ideal for a hearty lunch on chilly days. It's a tasty and filling meal that's high in vitamins, minerals, and antioxidants.

Serving Size: Four servings

Prep time: 15 minutes.

Cook time: 30 minutes.

Ingredients:

- 1 tablespoon of olive oil.

- One onion, chopped

- 3 garlic cloves, minced

- One medium butternut squash, peeled, seeded, and chopped

- 4 cups veggie broth.

- 1 teaspoon dried thyme.

- Half a teaspoon of crushed cinnamon

- Add salt and pepper to taste.

- Serve with Greek yogurt or coconut cream (optional).

Instructions:

1. In a large pot, warm the olive oil over medium heat. Cook the diced onion and garlic for about 5 minutes, or until softened.

2. Add the chopped butternut squash, vegetable broth, dried thyme, ground cinnamon, salt, and pepper to the pot.

3. Bring to a boil, then reduce to a low heat and cook for 20-25 minutes, until the butternut squash is soft.

4. Using an immersion blender, purée the soup until smooth. Alternatively, transfer the soup in stages to a blender and purée until smooth before returning to the pot.
5. Taste and adjust seasonings as necessary.
6. Serve the butternut squash soup hot, topped with a dollop of Greek yogurt or coconut cream, if desired.

Teriyaki Tofu Bowl

This teriyaki tofu dish is a delicious and filling lunch choice full of plant-based protein and nutritious ingredients. It's simple to make with your favorite vegetables and grains for a nutritious supper.

Serving Size: Two servings

Prep time: 15 minutes.

Cook time: 20 minutes.

Ingredients:

- 1 block of extra firm tofu, pressed and cubed

- 1/4 cup low-sodium soy sauce or tamari.

- Two teaspoons of honey or maple syrup

- 1 tablespoon of rice vinegar.

- 1 teaspoon of sesame oil.

- 2 garlic cloves, minced

- 1 teaspoon of grated ginger.

- 2 cups cooked brown rice or quinoa.

- 2 cups of mixed veggies (broccoli, bell peppers, snap peas).

- 1 tablespoon of sesame seeds for garnish.

- Sliced green onions for garnish.

Instructions:

1. In a small mixing bowl, combine the soy sauce or tamari, honey or maple syrup, rice vinegar, sesame oil, minced garlic, and grated ginger to make the teriyaki sauce.

2. In a large skillet or wok, heat 1 tablespoon oil over medium heat.

3. Cook the cubed tofu for 5-7 minutes, until golden brown and crispy on all sides.

4. Toss the tofu in the skillet with the teriyaki sauce until well coated.

5. Cook for another 2-3 minutes, or until the sauce thickens and the tofu is evenly coated.

6. In a separate skillet, cook the mixed vegetables until tender-crisp.

7. To make the bowls, split the cooked brown rice or quinoa into two bowls.

8. Top with teriyaki tofu and stir-fried veggies.

9. Before serving, garnish with sesame seeds and thinly sliced green onions.

Turkey and Cheese Roll-ups

These turkey and cheese roll-ups are a simple but filling lunch alternative that's ideal for on-the-go. They're a quick and easy way to keep energized and focused throughout the day, thanks to their high protein content and minimal carbohydrates.

Serving Size: Two servings

Prep time: 5 minutes.

Cooking time: 0 minutes.

Ingredients:

- 4 slices of deli turkey breast.
- Two pieces of cheese (either cheddar, Swiss, or your favorite)
- 1/4 cup young spinach leaves.
- One tablespoon mustard or mayonnaise

Instructions:

1. Place the turkey slices flat on a clean surface.
2. Place one piece of cheese on top of each turkey slice.
3. Spread mustard or mayonnaise equally on the cheese.
4. Spread a few young spinach leaves on top of the mustard or mayonnaise.
5. Roll each turkey slice tightly to create a roll-up.
6. Cut the roll-ups in half diagonally and place them in a container for a portable lunch.

Chapter 5: Healthy Dinners for Blood Sugar Control

Baked Lemon Herb Salmon

This baked lemon herb salmon is flavorful and high in protein and omega-3 fatty acids. It's a light and refreshing dinner choice suitable for either a weeknight or a special occasion.

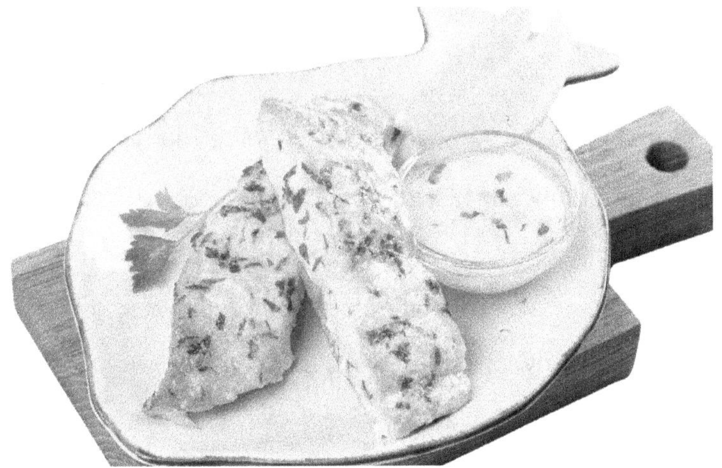

Serving Size: Four servings

Prep time: 10 minutes.

Cook time: 15 minutes.

Ingredients:

- 4 Salmon fillets

- 2 tablespoons olive oil.

- 2 garlic cloves, minced

- Zest and juice of one lemon

- 1 tablespoon of chopped fresh parsley.

- 1 teaspoon of dried dill.

- Add salt and pepper to taste.

- Lemon slices as garnish.

Instructions:

1. Preheat the oven to 400 °F (200 °C). Line a baking sheet with parchment paper.

2. In a small mixing bowl, combine olive oil, minced garlic, lemon zest, lemon juice, chopped parsley, dried dill, salt, and pepper.

3. Place the salmon fillets on the prepared baking sheet.

4. Brush the lemon herb mixture over the salmon fillets to coat them evenly.

5. Bake in the preheated oven for 12-15 minutes, or until the salmon is fully cooked and readily flaked with a fork.

6. Remove from the oven and garnish with lemon slices before serving.

7. Serve the baked lemon herb salmon hot alongside your favorite side dishes.

Roasted Garlic and Parmesan Brussels sprouts

These roasted garlic parmesan Brussels sprouts are crunchy, savory, and flavorful. They make a fantastic side dish or vegetarian main meal for a nutritious dinner.

Serving Size: Four servings
Prep time: 10 minutes.
Cook time: 25 minutes.

Ingredients:

- 1 pound of Brussels sprouts, cut and halved
- 2 tablespoons olive oil.

- 4 garlic cloves, minced
- 1/4 cup grated parmesan cheese.
- Add salt and pepper to taste.

Instructions:

1. Preheat the oven to 400 °F (200 °C). Line a baking sheet with parchment paper.
2. In a large mixing bowl, combine the Brussels sprouts, olive oil, chopped garlic, grated Parmesan cheese, salt, and pepper.
3. Place the Brussels sprouts in a single layer on the prepared baking sheet.
4. Roast the Brussels sprouts in the preheated oven for 20-25 minutes, or until soft and caramelized, tossing halfway through.
5. Remove from the oven and place in a serving dish.
6. Roasted garlic parmesan Brussels sprouts are a tasty and nutritious side dish. Serve hot.

Lemon Garlic Shrimp Pasta

This lemon garlic shrimp pasta is a light and tasty dinner alternative that is quick and simple to make. It's a well-balanced dinner with protein from the shrimp and fiber from the whole wheat pasta that will keep you full without weighing you down.

Serving Size: Four servings

Prep time: 10 minutes.

Cook time: 15 minutes.

Ingredients:

- 8 ounces whole wheat spaghetti or linguine.
- 1 tablespoon of olive oil.
- To prepare, skin and devein 1 pound of large shrimp and mince 4 cloves of garlic.
- Zest and juice of one lemon
- 1/4 cup chopped fresh parsley.
- Add salt and pepper to taste.
- Grated Parmesan cheese for serving is optional.

Instructions:

1. Cook the whole wheat spaghetti or linguine according to the package directions, until al dente. Drain and set aside.

2. In a large skillet, heat the olive oil over medium heat. Cook the shrimp and minced garlic for 2-3 minutes per side, or until pink and opaque.

3. In the skillet with the shrimp, combine the cooked pasta, lemon zest, lemon juice, chopped parsley, salt, and pepper.

4. Toss until everything is evenly blended and heated thoroughly.

5. Remove from heat and serve the lemon garlic shrimp pasta hot, topped with grated Parmesan cheese if preferred.

Turkey and Vegetable Quinoa Skillet

This turkey and veggie quinoa skillet is a healthy and filling one-pot meal ideal for hectic weeknights. It's a well-balanced meal option that the whole family will like, thanks to its lean protein, nutritious grains, and abundant vegetables.

Serving Size: Four servings

Prep time: 10 minutes.

Cook time: 25 minutes.

Ingredients:

- 1 tablespoon of olive oil.
- One onion, chopped
- 2 garlic cloves, minced
- 1 pound of ground turkey.
- 1 cup of quinoa, rinsed
- 2 cups low-sodium chicken broth.
- 1 cup diced tomatoes, canned or fresh.
- 2 cups chopped veggies (carrots, zucchini, and bell peppers).
- 1 teaspoon of dried oregano.
- 1 teaspoon dried basil.
- Add salt and pepper to taste.
- Grated Parmesan cheese for serving is optional.

Instructions:

1. In a large skillet, heat the olive oil over medium heat. Cook for about 5 minutes, stirring in the diced onion and minced garlic.

2. Cook the ground turkey in the skillet, breaking it up with a spoon, until browned and well cooked.

3. Combine the quinoa, chicken broth, diced tomatoes, chopped veggies, dried oregano, dried basil, salt, and pepper.

4. Bring the mixture to a boil, then reduce to a low heat, cover, and simmer for 15-20 minutes, or until the quinoa is cooked and the liquid has been absorbed.

5. Remove from the heat and cover the skillet for 5 minutes before serving.

6. Serve the turkey and veggie quinoa skillet hot, garnished with grated Parmesan cheese as desired.

Baked Chicken Parmesan

This baked chicken Parmesan is a healthier take on the classic Italian dish, featuring delicate chicken breasts wrapped in a crispy breadcrumb crust and topped with marinara sauce and melting mozzarella cheese. It's a crowd-pleasing meal option that will quickly become a family favorite.

Serving Size: Four servings
Prep time: 15 minutes.
Cook time: 25 minutes.

Ingredients:

- 4 boneless and skinless chicken breasts.
- 1 cup of whole wheat breadcrumbs.
- Ingredients: 1/2 cup grated Parmesan cheese, 1 teaspoon dried oregano.
- 1 teaspoon dried basil.
- Add salt and pepper to taste.
- One egg, beaten
- 1 cup marinara sauce.

- 1 cup shredded mozzarella cheese.
- Chopped fresh basil for garnish is optional.

Instructions:

1. Preheat the oven to 400 °F (200 °C). Line a baking sheet with parchment paper.
2. In a shallow bowl, mix together the whole wheat breadcrumbs, grated Parmesan cheese, dried oregano, dried basil, salt, and pepper.
3. Dip each chicken breast in the beaten egg, then dredge in the breadcrumb mixture, gently pressing to adhere.
4. Place the coated chicken breasts on the prepared baking sheet.
5. Bake in a preheated oven for 20 minutes.
6. Remove the baking sheet from the oven and spread the marinara sauce over each chicken breast.
7. Top each chicken breast with shredded mozzarella cheese.
8. Return the baking sheet to the oven for an additional 5-7 minutes, or until the cheese is

melted and bubbling and the chicken is thoroughly cooked.

9. Take the chicken out of the oven and let it rest for a few minutes before serving.

10. If preferred, garnish with freshly chopped basil before serving.

Grilled Lemon Herb Chicken

This grilled lemon herb chicken is juicy, tasty, and ideal for a healthy meal. Marinated in a zesty blend of lemon, garlic, and herbs, this tasty and satisfying dinner is sure to become a family favorite.

Serving Size: Four servings

Prep time: 10 minutes.

Cook time: 15 minutes.

Ingredients:

- 4 boneless and skinless chicken breasts.
- 1/4 cup olive oil.
- Zest and juice of one lemon

- 2 garlic cloves, minced
- 1 tablespoon of chopped fresh herbs (such as rosemary, thyme, or parsley).
- Add salt and pepper to taste.
- Lemon slices as garnish.

Instructions:

1. To prepare the marinade, combine the olive oil, lemon zest, lemon juice, minced garlic, chopped fresh herbs, salt, and pepper in a small bowl.
2. Place the chicken breasts in a shallow dish or a sealable plastic bag.
3. Pour the marinade over the chicken and make sure it is well coated.
4. Marinate in the refrigerator for at least 30 minutes and up to 4 hours.
5. Preheat the grill for medium-high heat. Remove the chicken from the marinade, discarding any excess marinade.
6. Grill the chicken breasts for 6-7 minutes on each side, or until fully cooked and no longer pink in the center.

7. Let the chicken rest for a few minutes before serving.

8. If desired, garnish with lemon slices before serving.

Garlic-Herb Roasted Vegetables

These garlic herb roasted vegetables are a beautiful and savory side dish that complements any main course. They're simple to make and full of flavor, thanks to a garlic herb marinade and a range of seasonal vegetables.

Serving Size: Four servings

Prep time: 10 minutes.

Cook time: 25 minutes.

Ingredients:

- 1 pound of mixed vegetables (carrots, bell peppers, zucchini, and cherry tomatoes)
- 2 tablespoons olive oil.
- 4 garlic cloves, minced
- 1 teaspoon dried thyme.

- 1 teaspoon dried rosemary.

- Add salt and pepper to taste.

- Fresh parsley for garnish (optional)

Instructions:

- Preheat the oven to 400 °F (200 °C). Line a baking sheet with parchment paper.

- Wash and chop the mixed vegetables into bite-sized pieces as needed.

- In a large mixing bowl, combine the veggies, olive oil, minced garlic, dried thyme, dried rosemary, salt, and pepper.

- Place the seasoned vegetables in a single layer on the prepared baking sheet.

- Roast the vegetables in the preheated oven for 20-25 minutes, or until soft and gently browned.

- Stir halfway through.

- Remove from the oven and place the roasted veggies in a serving dish.

- Garnish with fresh parsley before serving.

Veggie-packed Spaghetti Bolognese

This veggie-packed spaghetti Bolognese is a healthy take on a traditional Italian dish. It's a full and satisfying supper that the entire family will enjoy, thanks to lean ground turkey, loads of vegetables, and a thick tomato sauce.

Serving Size: Four servings

Prep time: 15 minutes.

Cook time: 30 minutes.

Ingredients:

- 8 ounces whole wheat spaghetti
- 1 tablespoon of olive oil.
- Dice one onion, two carrots, and two celery stalks. Mince two cloves of garlic.
- 1 pound of lean ground turkey.
- 1 (14.5 oz) can of diced tomatoes.
- 1 cup of tomato sauce.
- 1 teaspoon of dried oregano.
- 1 teaspoon dried basil.

- Add salt and pepper to taste.
- Grated Parmesan cheese for serving is optional.

Instructions:

1. Cook whole wheat spaghetti according to package directions until al dente.
2. Drain and set aside.
3. In a large skillet, heat the olive oil over medium heat.
4. Cook for about 5 minutes, stirring in the diced onion, carrots, celery, and minced garlic.
5. Cook the lean ground turkey in the skillet, breaking it up with a spoon, until browned and thoroughly done.
6. Combine the diced tomatoes, tomato sauce, dried oregano, dried basil, salt, and pepper.
7. Simmer the Bolognese sauce for 15-20 minutes, stirring occasionally, until it thickens and the flavors blend.
8. Serve the veggie-packed spaghetti Bolognese over cooked whole wheat spaghetti, garnished with grated Parmesan cheese, as desired.

Quinoa & Black Bean Skillet

This quinoa and black bean skillet is a flavorful and nutritious one-pot meal that is quick and simple to make. It's a nutritious dinner option that's ideal for busy weeknights, thanks to its high protein, fiber, and vegetable content.

Serving Size: Four servings
Prep time: 10 minutes.
Cook time: 25 minutes.

Ingredients:

- 1 tablespoon of olive oil.
- One onion, chopped
- To prepare, mince 2 garlic cloves, dice 1 bell pepper, and dice 1 zucchini.
- 1 cup corn kernels, fresh or frozen
- One (15 oz) can of black beans, drained and rinsed
- 1 cup of quinoa, rinsed

- 2 cups vegetable broth and 1 teaspoon chili powder.
- 1/2 teaspoon of ground cumin
- Add salt and pepper to taste.
- Fresh cilantro for garnish (optional)

Instructions:

1. In a large skillet, heat the olive oil over medium heat. Cook for about 5 minutes, stirring in the diced onion and minced garlic.
2. Add the diced bell pepper, zucchini, and corn kernels to the skillet. Cook for 5 more minutes, or until the vegetables are tender.
3. Combine the black beans, rinsed quinoa, vegetable broth, chili powder, ground cumin, salt, and pepper.
4. Bring the mixture to a boil, then reduce to a low heat, cover, and simmer for 15-20 minutes, or until the quinoa is cooked and the liquid has been absorbed.
5. Remove from the heat and cover the skillet for 5 minutes before serving.

6. Garnish with fresh cilantro before serving.

Turkey and Vegetable Stir-Fry

This turkey and vegetable stir-fry is a quick and flavorful dinner option ideal for busy weeknights. It's a nutritious meal that the whole family will enjoy, thanks to its lean protein and abundance of vegetables.

Serving Size: Four servings
Prep time: 15 minutes.
Cook time: 15 minutes.

Ingredients:
- 1 tablespoon of olive oil.
- 1 pound of ground turkey.
- 1 onion, thinly sliced
- 2 bell peppers, thinly sliced
- 1 zucchini, thinly sliced
- 1 cup snap peas
- 1/4 cup low-sodium soy sauce or tamari.
- 2 tablespoons hoisin sauce

- 1 tablespoon of rice vinegar.
- 2 garlic cloves, minced
- 1 teaspoon of grated ginger.
- 2 green onions, thinly sliced
- Cooked brown rice for serving

Instructions:

1. In a large skillet or wok, heat the olive oil over medium heat.
2. Add the ground turkey and cook, breaking it up with a spoon, until browned and cooked through.
3. Add the thinly sliced onion, bell peppers, zucchini, and snap peas to the skillet. Cook for 5-7 minutes, or until the vegetables are tender-crisp.
4. In a small bowl, whisk together the low-sodium soy sauce or tamari, hoisin sauce, rice vinegar, chopped garlic, and grated ginger.
5. Pour the sauce over the turkey and veggies in the skillet.
6. Stir to coat everything evenly and simmer for a further 2-3 minutes.

7. Remove from the heat and garnish with thinly
   sliced green onions.

8. Serve the turkey and vegetable stir-fry hot over
   cooked brown rice.

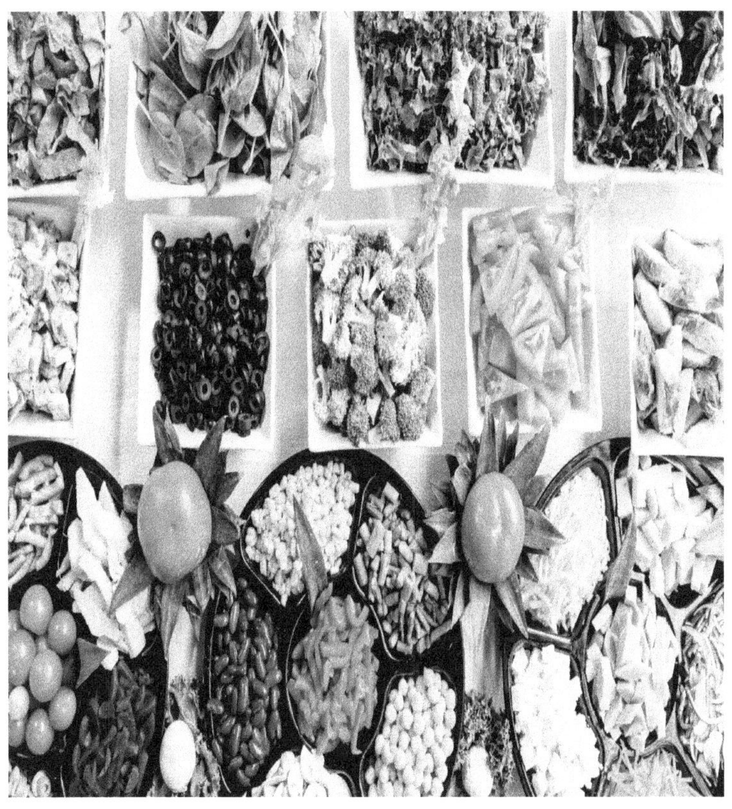

Chapter 6: Snacks and Treats for Balanced Blood Glucose

Greek Yogurt Parfait

This Greek yogurt parfait is a simple but filling snack that is ideal for any time of day. Layers of creamy Greek yogurt, fresh fruit, and crunchy granola make for a well-balanced snack rich in protein, fiber, and critical nutrients.

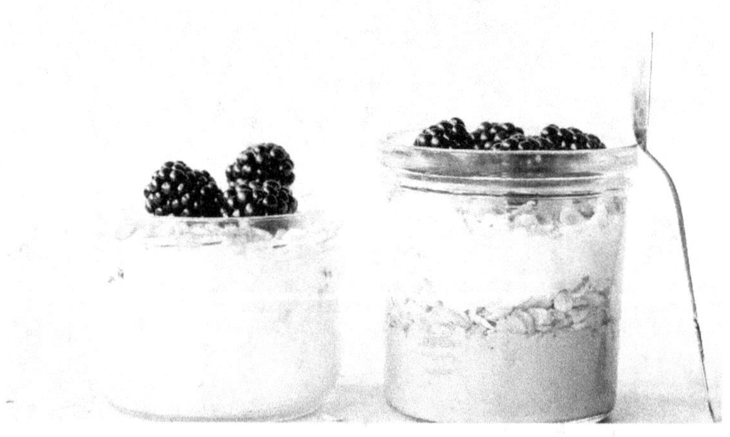

Serving Size: One parfait.

Prep time: 5 minutes.

Ingredients:

- 1/2 cup Greek yogurt.

- 1/4 cup mixed berries (strawberries, blueberries and raspberries)

- 2 tbsp granola.

- ***Optional:*** drizzle with honey or maple syrup.

Instructions:

- In a glass or dish, combine the Greek yogurt, mixed berries, and granola.

- Repeat the layers until all ingredients have been utilized, finishing with a sprinkling of granola on top.

- Drizzle with honey or maple syrup as desired.

- Serve immediately and enjoy this delicious and nutritious Greek yogurt parfait.

Apple slices with almond butter

This simple snack combines crisp apple slices with creamy almond butter for a pleasing blend of sweetness and crunch. It's a nutritious snack that contains fiber, protein, and healthy fats to keep you full and energized in between meals.

Serving Size: One serving
Prep time: 5 minutes.

Ingredients:

- 1 sliced apple
- and 2 tablespoons of almond butter.

Instructions:

1. Place the apple slices on a platter or serving dish.
2. Pour the almond butter into a small bowl or ramekin for dipping.
3. Dip the apple slices into the almond butter and enjoy this tasty and nutritious snack.

Dark Chocolate Avocado Mousse

This delectable yet healthier dessert combines ripe avocados and dark chocolate for a creamy, luscious delight. It is naturally sweet and high in heart-healthy lipids, antioxidants, and fiber.

Serving Size: Four servings

Prep time: 10 minutes.

Cooking time: 0 minutes.

Ingredients:

- Two ripe avocados, peeled and pitted.
- 1/4 cup cocoa powder.
- 1/4 cup honey or maple syrup.
- Ingredients: 1 teaspoon vanilla extract, pinch of salt.
- 1/4 cup unsweetened almond or coconut milk.
- Dark chocolate shavings for garnish are optional.

Instructions:

1. In a food processor or blender, combine ripe avocados, chocolate powder, maple syrup or honey, vanilla extract, salt, and almond milk.
2. Blend until smooth and creamy, scraping the sides of the bowl as necessary.

3. Divide the avocado mousse across serving dishes or glasses.

4. Place in the fridge for at least 30 minutes before serving.

5. Garnish with dark chocolate shavings before serving.

6. This rich and creamy dark chocolate avocado mousse makes an excellent guilt-free dessert or sweet treat.

Trail Mix Energy Bites

These trail mix energy bites are filled with nuts, seeds, dried fruit, and oats, making them a nutritious and portable snack. They're simple to create and may be filled with your favorite ingredients for unlimited variety.

Serving size: 12 bites.

Prep time: 10 minutes.

Cooking time: 0 minutes.

Ingredients:

- 1 cup rolled oats.

- 1/2 cup nut butter (almond, peanut, or cashew)

- 1/4 cup honey or maple syrup.

- 1/4 cup chopped nuts (such as almonds, walnuts, or pecans)

- Add 1/4 cup chopped dry fruit (raisins, cranberries, or apricots) and 2 tablespoons seeds (sunflower, pumpkin, or chia).

- 1 teaspoon of vanilla extract.

- Pinch of salt.

Instructions:

1. In a large mixing bowl, mix together the rolled oats, nut butter, honey or maple syrup, chopped nuts, dried fruit, seeds, vanilla essence, and salt.

2. Stir together all of the ingredients until they create a sticky dough.

3. Roll the dough into little 1 inch balls and place on a parchment-lined baking pan.

4. Place the trail mix energy bites in the refrigerator for at least 30 minutes before serving.

5. Refrigerate any leftovers in an airtight container for up to a week.

6. Enjoy these nutritious and delicious trail mix energy bites as a quick snack on the run.

Cucumber and Hummus Bites

These cucumber and hummus bites are a pleasant and filling snack that is ideal for soothing cravings in between meals. For a nutritious and savory treat, combine crisp cucumber slices with creamy hummus and garnish with your favorite toppings.

Serving Size: One serving

Prep time: 5 minutes.

Ingredients:

- 1 cucumber sliced into rounds.
- 2 tablespoons hummus.
- Optional garnishes include cherry tomatoes, chopped olives, and fresh herbs.

Instructions:

1. Place the cucumber slices on a serving dish or plate.
2. Spoon a tiny amount of hummus onto each cucumber slice.
3. Garnish with cherry tomatoes, sliced olives, or fresh herbs if preferred.
4. These cool cucumber and hummus bites make a great snack.

Guacamole-topped vegetable sticks

This snack blends crunchy veggie sticks with creamy guacamole for a tasty and healthful treat. It's an excellent choice for filling hunger between meals, as it's high in vitamins, minerals, and healthy fats.

Serving Size: One serving
Prep time: 10 minutes.

Ingredients:

- Assorted vegetable sticks (carrots, celery, bell peppers, and cucumber)
- 1 ripe avocado.
- Juice half a lime and add 1/4 teaspoon garlic powder.
- Add salt and pepper to taste.

Instructions:

1. Wash and cut the veggie sticks into strips.
2. In a separate bowl, mash the ripe avocado with lime juice, garlic powder, salt, and pepper to make guacamole.
3. Serve the veggie sticks beside the guacamole for dipping.
4. Enjoy this nutritious and enjoyable snack high in vitamins and healthy fats.

Cottage Cheese and Pineapple Cups

These cottage cheese and pineapple cups are a protein-rich and pleasant snack that will satisfy your hunger in between meals. For a tasty and healthful treat, combine juicy pineapple chunks with creamy cottage cheese.

Serving Size: One serving

Prep time: 5 minutes.

Ingredients:

- 1/2 cup cottage cheese.
- 1/2 cup pineapple pieces, fresh or canned.
- Fresh mint leaves for garnish (optional).

Instructions:

1. Divide the cottage cheese evenly into serving cups or bowls.
2. Top each cup with pineapple slices.
3. Garnish with fresh mint leaves if preferred.
4. Serve immediately and enjoy this protein-rich snack.

Banana Oatmeal Cookies

These banana oatmeal cookies are a healthier alternative to typical cookies, including no added sugar and plenty of natural sweetness from ripe bananas. They're simple to create and ideal for fulfilling sweet cravings without causing guilt.

Serving size: 12 cookies.
Prep time: 10 minutes.
Cook time: 15 minutes.

Ingredients:

- Two ripe bananas, mashed
- 1 cup rolled oats.
- 1/4 cup chopped nuts or seeds (such pumpkin seeds, almonds, or walnuts)
- 1/4 cup raisins or dried cranberries.
- 1/2 teaspoon of cinnamon.
- 1/4 teaspoon of vanilla extract.

Instructions:

1. Preheat the oven to 350° Fahrenheit (175° Celsius).

2. Line a baking sheet with parchment paper.

3. In a mixing bowl, add mashed bananas, rolled oats, chopped nuts or seeds, raisins or dried cranberries, cinnamon, and vanilla essence.

4. Drop spoonfuls of the cookie dough onto the prepared baking sheet, spacing them evenly.

5. Use a spoon or fork to softly flatten each biscuit.

6. Bake the cookies in a preheated oven for 15-18 minutes, or until golden brown and firm to touch.

7. Remove from the oven and let the cookies cool on the baking sheet for a few minutes before moving to a wire rack to finish cooling.

8. Enjoy these banana oatmeal cookies as a healthy and filling sweet snack.

Energy-Boosting Smoothie Packs

These energy-boosting smoothie packets are ideal for hectic mornings or quick snacks on the run. Simply combine the frozen smoothie ingredients with your preferred liquid for a healthful and pleasant snack anytime, anyplace.

Serving Size: One smoothie pack.

Prep time: 10 minutes.

Ingredients:

- 1/2 cup mixed berries (strawberries, blueberries and raspberries)
- 1/2 banana, cut.
- 1/4 cup spinach leaves.
- 1 tbsp chia or flaxseeds
- 1/4 cup Greek yogurt (optional).
- 1/2 cup coconut water or almond milk.
- 1/2 cup ice cubes.

Instructions:

1. In a small resealable plastic bag or container, combine the mixed berries, sliced banana, spinach leaves, chia seeds or flaxseeds, and Greek yogurt (if using).

2. Seal the bag or container and freeze until ready for use.

3. When you're ready to prepare the smoothie, add the frozen smoothie pack contents to a blender.

4. Combine the coconut water or almond milk with the ice cubes.

5. Blend until smooth and creamy, adding additional liquid as needed to achieve the desired consistency.

6. Pour the smoothie into a glass and enjoy this energizing snack on the run.

Almond Butter Stuffed Dates

These almond butter-stuffed dates are a sweet and satisfying snack that can help you curb cravings. Sweet Medjool dates are filled with creamy almond butter for a delectable blend of flavors and textures.

Serving Size: One serving

Prep time: 5 minutes.

Ingredients:

- Pit 6 Medjool dates and add 2 tablespoons almond butter.
- Optional toppings include chopped nuts, shredded coconut, and dark chocolate chips.

Instructions:

1. Carefully cut each Medjool date lengthwise and remove the pit.
2. Fill each date with a tablespoon of almond butter.
3. Sprinkle with chopped nuts, shredded coconut, or dark chocolate chips if desired.
4. Serve these almond butter stuffed dates immediately for a pleasant and nutritious snack.

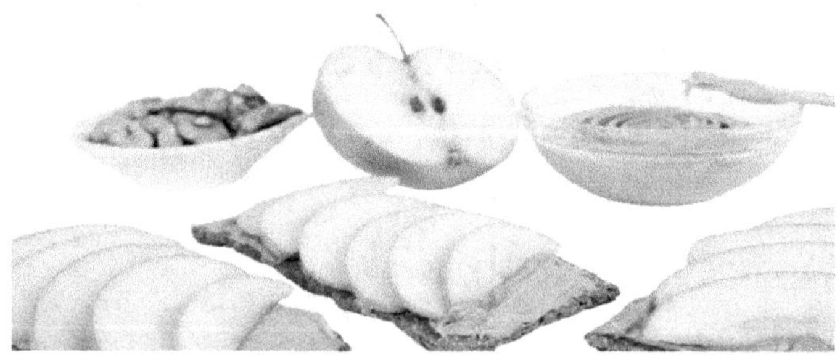

Chapter 7: Drinks for Hydration and Blood Sugar Control

Citrus-infused water

Staying hydrated is critical for managing diabetes, and this citrus-infused water offers a delicious twist to regular water. It's a hydrating beverage full of vitamin C and antioxidants from fresh citrus fruits, making it ideal for any time of day.

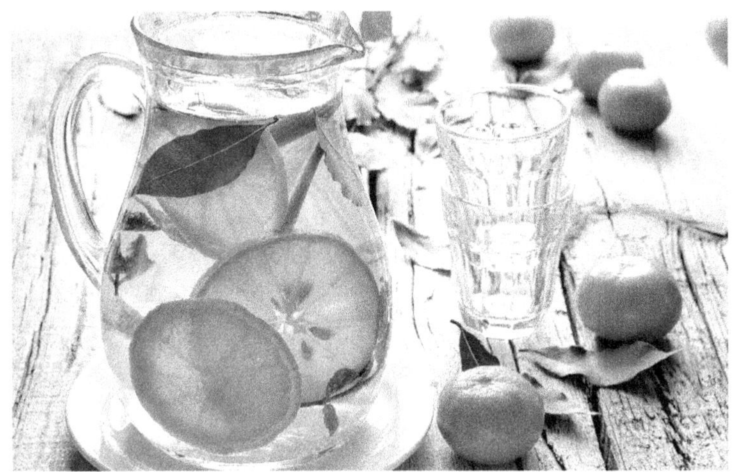

Serving Size: One serving

Prep time: 5 minutes.

Ingredients:

- One lemon, thinly sliced
- Ingredients: 1 thinly sliced lime, 1 orange, and 2 sprigs of fresh mint.
- 4 cups of water.
- Ice cubes (Optional)

Instructions:

1. In a large pitcher, combine the thinly sliced lemon, lime, and oranges.
2. Include the fresh mint sprigs.
3. Fill the pitcher with water and gently whisk until combined.
4. Refrigerate for at least an hour to allow the flavors to combine.
5. If desired, you can serve the citrus-infused water over ice.
6. Drink this pleasant and hydrating beverage throughout the day.

Cucumber-Mint Cooler

This cucumber mint cooler is a pleasant and hydrating beverage that is naturally low in sugar. Cucumber gives hydration, and fresh mint adds taste. It's the ideal drink for hot summer days or whenever you need a refreshing pick-up.

Serving Size: One serving

Prep time: 5 minutes.

Ingredients:

- 1/2 cucumber, sliced.
- 4–5 fresh mint leaves
- 1 cup of sparkling water.
- Ice cubes
- Optional garnishes include thin cucumber slices and mint sprigs.

Instructions:

1. In a tumbler, muddle the sliced cucumber and fresh mint leaves to release their flavors.

2. Fill the glass with ice cubes.

3. Pour the sparkling water over the ice and cucumber-mint mixture.

4. Stir gently to mix.

5. Garnish with thin cucumber slices and mint sprigs if preferred.

6. Serve immediately and enjoy the delicious cucumber mint cooler.

Ginger Turmeric Tea

This ginger turmeric tea is a warming and immune-boosting beverage that is ideal for promoting general wellness. Ginger and turmeric are anti-inflammatory and antioxidant-rich, making this tea a relaxing and pleasant beverage at any time of day.

Serving Size: One serving

Prep time: 5 minutes.

Cooking time: 10 minutes.

Ingredients:

- 1 inch of freshly sliced fresh ginger.
- 1 teaspoon ground turmeric.
- 2 glasses of water.
- One tablespoon honey (optional)
- Fresh lemon slices for garnish (optional).

Instructions:

1. In a small saucepan, mix together the thinly sliced ginger, ground turmeric, and water.
2. Bring the mixture to a simmer over medium heat.
3. Reduce the heat to low and let the tea simmer for 10 minutes to allow the flavors to combine.
4. Remove from the heat and drain the tea into a mug.
5. If desired, stir in honey.
6. Garnish with fresh lemon slices if preferred.
7. Serve hot and enjoy this calming ginger turmeric tea.

Berry Green Smoothie

This berry green smoothie has vitamins, minerals, and antioxidants from leafy greens and mixed berries. It's a delicious and nutritious way to start the day or refuel after a workout, and the sugar amount is balanced to help with blood sugar regulation.

Serving Size: One serving
Prep time: 5 minutes.

Ingredients:

- 1 cup of spinach or kale leaves.
- 1/2 cup mixed berries (strawberries, blueberries and raspberries)
- 1/2 banana.
- 1/2 cup unsweetened almond milk or coconut water.
- 1 tbsp chia or flaxseeds
- Ice cubes

Instructions:

1. In a blender, combine spinach or kale leaves, mixed berries, banana, almond milk or coconut water, and chia or flaxseeds.
2. Blend until smooth and creamy, adding additional liquid as needed to achieve the desired consistency.
3. Add the ice cubes and mix again until smooth.
4. Pour the berry-green smoothie into a glass and serve immediately.
5. Enjoy this healthful and well-balanced smoothie as a delightful snack or dinner alternative.

Coconut water electrolyte drink

This coconut water electrolyte drink is a natural and hydrating beverage that replaces key minerals lost through sweating. It's a refreshing and delicious way to stay hydrated during exercise or in hot weather, with no added sugars.

Serving Size: One serving

Prep time: 5 minutes.

Ingredients:

- 1 cup coconut water.
- Juice from 1/2 lime.
- Add a pinch of sea salt and ice cubes.

Instructions:

1. In a glass, mix together the coconut water and lime juice.
2. Add a pinch of sea salt and mix until dissolved.
3. Fill the glass with ice cubes.
4. Stir gently to mix.
5. Serve immediately and enjoy this delightful coconut water electrolyte drink.

Iced green tea with mint and lemon

This iced green tea with mint and lemon is a delicious, low-sugar beverage ideal for hot summer days. Green tea is high in antioxidants and provides a modest energy boost, while fresh mint and lemon create a refreshing flavor.

Serving Size: One serving

Prep time: 10 minutes.

Cook time: 5 minutes.

Ingredients:

- One green tea bag.
- 1 cup water.
- Fresh mint leaves with lemon slices.
- Ice cubes

Instructions:

1. In a small saucepan, heat 1 cup of water until it boils.
2. Remove from the heat and add the green tea bag.
3. Steep for 3-5 minutes, then take out the tea bag and allow it cool to room temperature.
4. Once the tea has cooled, put it to an ice-filled glass.
5. Place fresh mint leaves and lemon slices in the glass.
6. Stir gently to mix.

7. Serve right away and enjoy this delightful iced green tea with mint and lemon.

Chamomile Lavender Tea

This chamomile lavender tea is a peaceful and calming beverage that can help you relax and relieve tension. Chamomile and lavender have natural calming characteristics, so this tea is great for relaxing in the evening.

Serving Size: One serving
Prep time: 5 minutes.
Cook time: 5 minutes.

Ingredients:

- One chamomile tea bag.
- 1 teaspoon of dried lavender flowers.
- 1 cup water.
- Honey or Stevia (optional)

Instructions:

1. In a small saucepan, heat 1 cup of water until it boils.

2. Remove from the fire and add the chamomile tea bag and dried lavender flowers.

3. Steep for 3-5 minutes, then remove the tea bag and filter out the lavender flowers.

4. For sweetness, add honey or stevia as desired.

5. Enjoy this calming chamomile lavender tea while it is still hot.

Pineapple Ginger Turmeric Smoothie

This pineapple ginger turmeric smoothie is a tropical and immune-boosting beverage full of vitamins, minerals, and antioxidants. Pineapple adds sweetness, and ginger and turmeric have anti-inflammatory properties.

Serving Size: One serving

Prep time: 5 minutes.

Ingredients:

- 1 cup of frozen pineapple pieces.

- 1/2 inch fresh ginger, peeled
- 1/2 teaspoon of ground turmeric.
- 1/2 cup unsweetened coconut milk.
- 1/4 cup Greek yogurt.
- Honey or maple syrup is optional.

Instructions:

1. In a blender, add frozen pineapple chunks, fresh ginger, ground turmeric, coconut milk, and Greek yogurt.
2. Blend until smooth and creamy, adding additional coconut milk as needed to achieve the desired consistency.
3. If you like it sweeter, add some honey or maple syrup.
4. Place the pineapple ginger turmeric smoothie in a glass and serve immediately.
5. Enjoy this tropical and immune-boosting smoothie as a healthy snack or lunch alternative.

Mocktail Mojito

This mocktail mojito is a pleasant and alcohol-free variation of the traditional cocktail, ideal for diabetics or anybody searching for a refreshing non-alcoholic beverage. Fresh mint, lime, and sparkling water combine for a refreshing and tasty beverage.

Serving Size: One serving

Prep time: 5 minutes.

Ingredients:

- 1/2 lime, sliced into wedges
- 4–5 fresh mint leaves
- One teaspoon of honey or stevia (optional)
- Sparkling water
- Ice cubes

Instructions:

1. In a glass, muddle the lime wedges and fresh mint leaves to release their flavors.
2. For sweetness, add honey or stevia as desired.

3. Fill the glass with ice cubes.

4. Pour sparkling water over the ice-lime mint mixture.

5. Stir gently to mix.

6. Garnish with a sprig of fresh mint.

7. Serve immediately and enjoy this cool mocktail mojito.

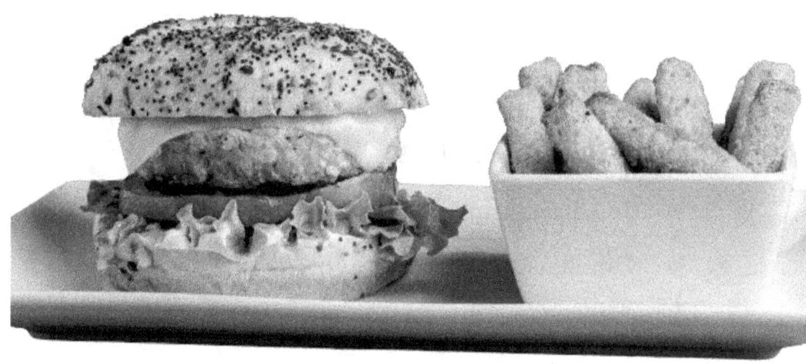

Chapter 8: Special Occasions and Holidays

Celebrating special milestones and holidays is an important part of life, but for people with type 2 diabetes, these celebrations can pose problems in terms of food choices and social interactions. In this chapter, we look at methods and recipes to help you negotiate these occasions with confidence while still enjoying wonderful meals and sweets.

Plan Diabetes-Friendly Parties and Gatherings

Hosting a Diabetes-Friendly Gathering

Planning a diabetic-friendly party or gathering requires careful consideration of meal options and serving sizes. Choose nutrient-dense, low-glycemic foods such as lean proteins, veggies, whole grains, and healthy fats. Provide a variety of dishes to meet diverse dietary needs and constraints. Keep guests interested and active by providing lots of water and unsweetened beverages, as well as encouraging physical exercise.

Holiday Meal Strategy

Navigating Holiday Meals with Type II Diabetes

Holiday meals sometimes include rich, delicious delicacies that may not be compatible with diabetes treatment goals. To successfully navigate holiday meals, adopt portion management and mindful eating. Fill your plate with non-starchy veggies, lean proteins, and whole grains, while limiting high-carbohydrate and high-sugar items. Keep moving throughout the day to help stabilize blood sugar levels, and bring a diabetes-friendly cuisine to share with family and friends.

Festive Desserts and Treats

Healthier Holiday Dessert Alternatives

Indulging in Christmas cakes and treats is part of the enjoyment, but it's critical to make wise decisions to control blood sugar levels. Choose sweets that contain whole grains, natural sweeteners, and fruit, such as fruit salads, baked apples, or sugar-free pumpkin pie. Experiment with different flours and ingredients to make healthier versions of traditional holiday desserts while maintaining flavor.

Eating out with Type 2 Diabetes

Eating Out and Managing Type 2 Diabetes

Dining out can be difficult for those with type 2 diabetes, but with proper planning, it is possible to enjoy restaurant meals while staying on track with diabetes management goals. Research restaurant menus ahead of time, select dishes with lean proteins, vegetables, and whole grains, and request dietary changes. Practice portion control, avoid sugary beverages and desserts, and think about sharing meals or bringing leftovers home.

Navigating Social Situations With Confidence

Confidently navigating social situations

Social circumstances such as parties, meals, and gatherings can be daunting for those with type 2 diabetes, but with proper planning and confidence, it is possible to enjoy these occasions while prioritizing health. Prepare ahead of time by eating a balanced meal or snack, bringing diabetes-friendly items to share, and communicating your dietary needs to hosts or restaurant staff. Instead of focusing entirely on eating, spend time engaging with others and enjoying the company.

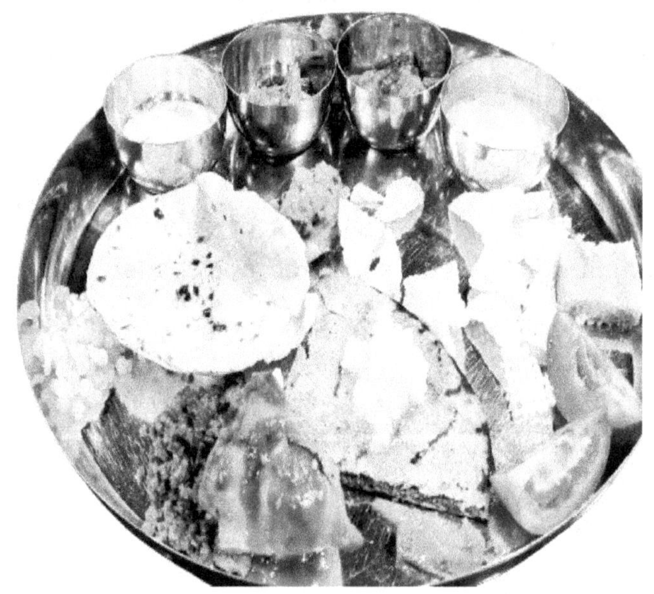

Chapter 9: BONUS 7-DAY Meal Planning for Type 2 Diabetes Management

Type 2 diabetes requires strict dietary management, including balanced meals that help maintain blood sugar levels. Here's a 7-day meal plan to help people with type 2 diabetes maintain stable blood glucose levels while eating delicious, satisfying meals.

Day 1:

Breakfast: Vegetable omelette prepared with eggs, spinach, bell peppers, and onions.

Whole grain toast.

unsweetened herbal tea or black coffee.

Lunch: Grilled chicken salad made with mixed greens, cherry tomatoes, cucumbers, and avocado

Balsamic vinaigrette dressing served on the side.

Dessert: Sliced apple.

Baked salmon fillet with lemon and herbs.

Quinoa pilaf and sautéed veggies

Steamed broccoli

Sparkling water with lemon as a beverage

Day 2:

Breakfast: Greek yogurt A parfait of plain Greek yogurt, mixed berries, and a sprinkle of chopped nuts.

Whole grain granola on top.

Green or herbal tea?

Lunch: Turkey and avocado wrap made with whole grain tortilla, sliced turkey breast, avocado, lettuce, and tomato

Carrot sticks with hummus for dip

Sparkling water with lime for beverages.

Dinner: Beef stir-fry with mixed veggies (broccoli, bell peppers, snap peas) in mild soy sauce.

Brown rice

On Day 3, we had sliced oranges as dessert

Breakfast: Overnight oats with rolled oats, almond milk, chia seeds, and a sprinkle of cinnamon

Sliced banana on top.

Unsweetened almond milk latte.

Lunch: Lentil soup with carrots, celery, onion, and spinach

Whole grain crackers on the side.

Dessert consists of mixed berries

Grilled tofu and teriyaki sauce

Roasted sweet potatoes.

Steamed green beans.

Sparkling water with cucumber as a beverage

Day 4:

Breakfast: Whole grain bread with mashed avocado and sliced tomatoes.

Optional toppings: poached egg, herbal tea, or black coffee

Lunch: Quinoa salad with chickpeas, chopped bell pepper, cucumber, and feta cheese.

Lemon vinaigrette dressing served on the side.

Apple slices with almond butter for dessert.

Dinner: Turkey meatballs with marinara sauce.

Zucchini noodles

Mixed green salad with lemon vinaigrette.

Unsweetened iced tea with lemon as a beverage

Breakfast: Vegetable and cheese scramble includes eggs, bell peppers, onions, and spinach.

Whole grain English muffins

Green or herbal tea?

Lunch: grilled shrimp skewers with lemon and garlic.

Quinoa tabbouleh salad with cucumber, tomatoes, parsley, and a lemon dressing.

Sparkling water with lime for beverages.

Dinner: Baked chicken breast with rosemary and thyme.

roasted Brussels sprouts with balsamic glaze.

Cauliflower mashed potatoes

Strawberry slices for dessert on Day 6

Breakfast: Smoothie with spinach, kale, banana, unsweetened almond milk, and a scoop of protein powder

Sprinkle some ground flaxseed on top.

unsweetened herbal tea or black coffee.

Lunch: Turkey and vegetable stir-fry with broccoli, bell peppers, and snap peas in a mild teriyaki sauce.

Brown rice

Dessert consists of mixed berries.

baked cod with lemon and herbs.

Quinoa pilaf served with roasted vegetables (zucchini, bell peppers, and onions).

Mixed green salad with balsamic vinaigrette.

Sparkling water with cucumber and mint for beverages.

Day 7:

Breakfast: Whole grain pancakes topped with Greek yogurt and mixed berries.

Drizzle with sugar-free maple syrup.

Green or herbal tea?

Lunch: Chickpea salad made with mixed greens, cherry tomatoes, cucumbers, and feta cheese

Lemon vinaigrette dressing served on the side.

Dessert option: sliced oranges.

Vegetable curry made with chickpeas, cauliflower, carrots, and spinach in coconut milk.

Brown rice

Sparkling water with lime for beverages.

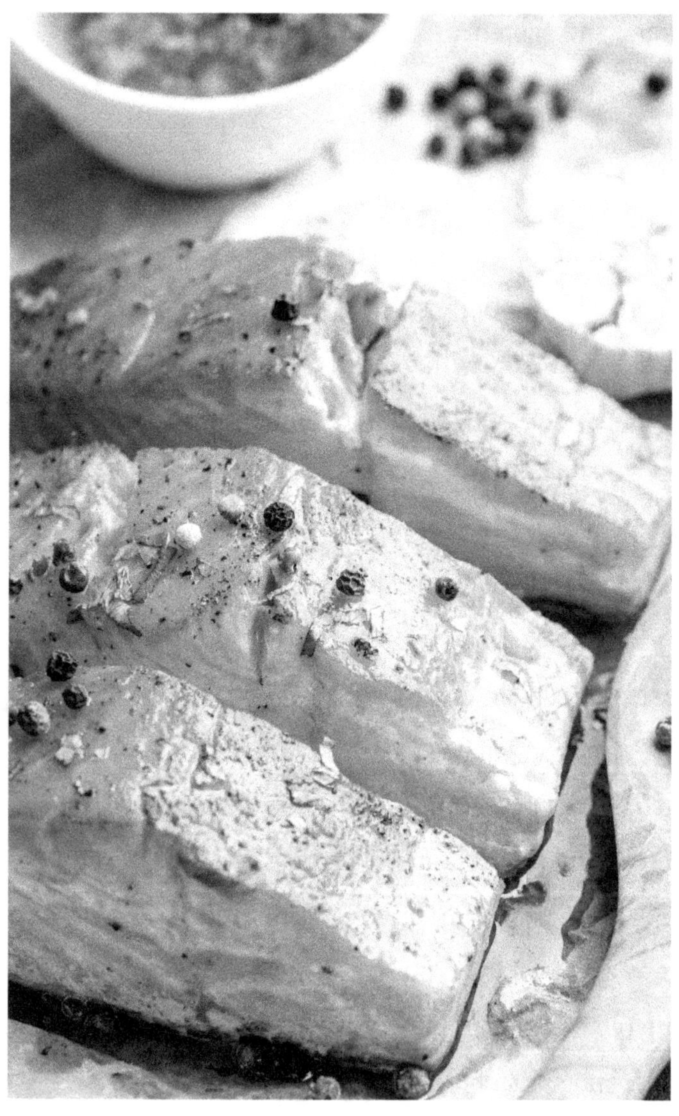

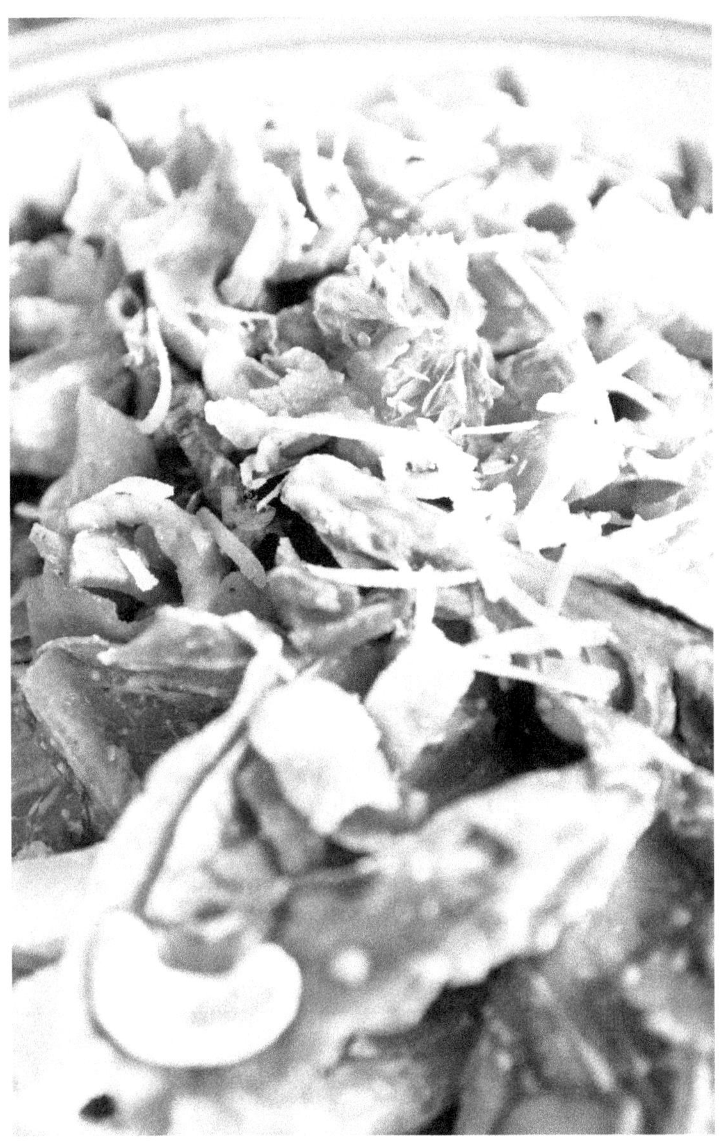

CONCLUSION

The Type 2 Diabetes Diet Cookbook is a thorough resource that teaches people with type 2 diabetes how to manage their health via eating. This cookbook has a wealth of knowledge, practical recommendations, and tasty dishes designed expressly to aid in blood sugar management and overall well-being.

The Type 2 Diabetes nutrition Cookbook is based on the concept that nutrition is essential for effectively controlling type 2 diabetes. Individuals who pay close attention to their food choices and portion amounts can stabilize blood sugar levels, lower the risk of problems, and enhance their general health. The cookbook opens with a thorough introduction of type 2 diabetes, explaining the disorder, its causes, risk factors, consequences, and the role of diet in disease management.

The Type 2 Diabetes Diet Cookbook places a strong emphasis on education and empowerment. Readers will learn important dietary principles for treating type 2 diabetes, including carbohydrate counting, glycemic index, portion control, and meal timing. With this information, people may make informed dietary decisions and create a tailored eating plan that meets their needs and tastes.

The cookbook has a wide range of tasty and diabetes-friendly recipes for every meal of the day, including breakfast, lunch, supper, snacks, and dessert. Each formulation is meticulously designed to deliver balanced nourishment while delighting the taste buds. From robust salads and delicious soups to fulfilling main courses and tempting desserts, the Type 2 Diabetes Diet Cookbook has something for everyone.

In addition to delicious dishes, the cookbook includes useful meal planning and preparation suggestions to help readers manage their dietary path with ease. Readers will learn how to plan and cook meals ahead of time, make informed grocery shopping decisions, and store and reheat meals properly. These helpful resources help people with type 2 diabetes enjoy delicious and nutritious meals while reducing stress and worry in the kitchen.

Additional resources

Additional resources on type 2 diabetes diets and cookbooks give vital assistance and information for people who want to control their condition properly through nutrition. These materials provide a variety of insights, recipes, and practical recommendations to help people with type 2 diabetes make more informed dietary decisions and enhance their overall health. Here are some suggested further resources:

The American Diabetes Association (ADA

The American Diabetes Association (ADA) provides a multitude of tools for managing type 2 diabetes, including dietary guidelines, meal planning guidance, and recipes.

Website: diabetes.org

The Diabetes Food Hub

The Diabetes Food Hub offers a selection of diabetes-friendly recipes, meal plans, and nutrition suggestions to help people with type 2 diabetes make healthier food choices.

Website: diabetesfoodhub.org.

Joslin Diabetes Center

The Joslin Diabetes Center provides teaching materials, cookbooks, and online resources for type 2 diabetes management, such as nutritional guidelines and meal planning tools.

Website: joslin.org.

The Diabetes Cookbook by Shasta Press

This cookbook has a variety of recipes designed exclusively for people with diabetes, delivering delicious and nutritious meal ideas to help with blood sugar management.

Book: The Diabetes Cookbook

The Type 2 Diabetes Cookbook and Meal Plan by Whitney English

A licensed dietitian wrote this cookbook, which includes a detailed meal plan and a range of recipes to assist people with type 2 diabetes eat properly and manage their disease efficiently.

Diabetes UK publishes The Type 2 Diabetes Cookbook and Meal Plan.

Diabetes UK offers a variety of information and support for people with diabetes, such as dietary guidance, recipe ideas, and meal planning tools.

Website: diabetes.org.uk

MyNetDiary

MyNetDiary is a complete software and website that provides tools for recording food intake, monitoring blood sugar levels, and setting tailored dietary goals for diabetics.

Website: mynetdiary.com.

The Diabetic News' cookbook, Eat Well with Diabetes,

This cookbook has a compilation of diabetes-friendly recipes, meal planning, and nutritional information to help diabetics make better eating choices.

Book: Eat Well With Diabetes Cookbook